An Easy Way
To Understand
Autism In Children

Also By Brian B Jacques

His very popular Series of Mini-Health Books includes:

- An Easy Way To Understand Eczema and Psoriasis
- An Easy Way To Understand Stress and Depression
- An Easy Way To Understand Vitamins and Minerals
- An Easy Way To Understand Parasites, Worms, Candida, Constipation & Detoxing
- An Easy Way To Understand Crohn's Disease and IBD
- An Easy Way To Understand Body Building For Men And Women
- An Easy Way To Understand Alzheimer's Disease
- An Easy Way To Understand Herpes
- An Easy Way To Understand Parkinson's Disease
- An Easy Way To Understand Autism In Children
- An Easy Way To Understand Fibromyalgia
- An Easy Way To Understand Your Body Systems
- An Easy Way To Understand Erectile Dysfunction
- An Easy Way To Understand Heart Disease, High Blood Pressure & Stroke
- An Easy Way To Understand Detoxing For Men & Women
- How To Lose Weight After 40
- How To Lose Weight And Maintain Your Ideal Weight Permanently
- Amino Acids & Enzymes—What Are They & Why Do You Need Them
- The Little A–Z Dictionary of Herbal Remedies
- The Magic Of Vitamins & Minerals
- Effective Methods To Stop Smoking
- Eat Wholefoods And Take Supplements—The Ultimate Lifestyle Guide
- Stress Busters Adult Coloring Book

All these books are available as Kindle Editions (available from the Kindle Store on Amazon.com, and other countries Amazon sites where the Kindle platform is supported.) Many of these books are also available for the Barnes and Noble "Nook". In addition, many of these titles are available as print editions from the Amazon website.

An Easy Way To Understand Autism In Children

Brian B Jacques

Wisdom For Life Media

ISBN - 13: 978-1546776826

ISBN - 10: 1546776826

Published in The United States of America.

"Education is the kindling of a flame, not the filling of a vessel." —Socrates

Contents

Acknowledgment

To the many people I have come into contact with throughout my life, whose belief in me has made everything possible and worthwhile.

1. A History of Autism

In the past it has been problematical to diagnose the symptoms of autism. In the beginning, sufferers were placed in psychiatric institutions and were hidden from society—in many cases for the rest of their lives.

We have to look to the early 1900s when a Swiss psychiatrist by the name of Eugen Bleuler first used the term to describe the behavior of adults with schizophrenia who demonstrated behavior that was not normally associated with schizophrenia. The patients that Eugen Bleuler described removed themselves from society and lived in their "own little world".

We then move to 1943, when Dr. Leo Kanner of Johns Hopkins University, gave a description of autism which was based on 11 children, who had withdrawn themselves from human contact from as early as one year of age. Their conditions included a lack of social interaction, being sensitive to sound, echolalia (repetition of a single word or phrase) and memory impairment.

In 1944 Hans Asperger (Asperger's syndrome was named after him) working independently of Kanner, wrote a paper concerning another group of children. In many ways they represented the children that Kanner was describing, the main difference being one of language. In the children Asperger was describing, there was no mention of echolalia, but a strange phenomenon as if it was like the children were talking as small adults. In addition, he also observed that their motor (nerve) activity was not as coordinated as would be found in normal children.

Additional work was being undertaken with children who had been potentially identified as being autistic. Bruno Bettelheim describes three sessions with children. He determined that their problems were "due to the emotional unavailability of their mothers".

In the years between the 1940s and 1960s many in the medical community had the belief that children who were being diagnosed as autistic were also schizophrenic—a common theory at this time that was blamed on bad parenting. This faulty diagnosis led to the result that many parents blamed themselves for their children's condition.

During the 1970s more information about autism began to spread to Sweden. In Sweden the children were termed autistic psychotic children. In the early 1980s, the Erica foundation began to offer programs of education and therapy to both the medical profession and parents.

The work of Hans Asperger remained relatively unknown until his book was translated into English in 1980. And unfortunately since the work of Kanner and Bettelheim often caused confusion, it became accepted practice to blame the mothers for their children's autistic diagnosis. The theory being that they were lacking in the ability to meet their children's emotional needs.

Researchers and doctors spent many years blaming what they termed exposure to a "frigid mother" for their children's language difficulties. Fortunately, these medical professionals ultimately realized that the children's disability was more complex than they first thought and that there was no single basic cause for the condition.

During the late 1980s autism research stepped up a pace and more physicians began to realize that neurological disturbances were the basic cause of autism. It became possible to group the many causes and symptoms that had been documented into categories, which at last, provided enough similarities to determine a single main diagnosis.

2. Causes

Quite a few theories have been investigated as to what causes autism. I have discussed some of these theories below, but at the present time, no one theory stands out from the rest as being the main cause. Autism is so complex that it is possible that there may be multiple triggers involved that when these are combined will cause someone to become autistic.

What is known is that autism is a disability that affects people's development and behavior skills in a variety of ways. It is important to understand that while the symptoms will vary between different individuals there is enough similarity for a definitive diagnosis to be given.

Let us now move on to the theories. One theory which is backed up by several case studies and is being discussed in parent and support groups is the possible link between children being immunized for measles and autism. In the case studies it has been determined that some children have a poor reaction to the preservatives that are used to dissolve the immunizing agent.

In reality the number of cases where children have been immunized and then go on to develop autism is quite small when compared to the total number of children who are diagnosed with autism. However, this theory is still being researched and the investigation is on-going. An unfortunate consequence of the research is that it is often funded by drug companies, who have a vested interest in ensuring that there is no link between immunization and autism.

Another theory is the possibility that there is a genetic link in that parents who have autism are more at risk of having children with autism than parents who do not have the condition. To date, no autistic gene has been identified that can be a cause of the syndrome.

As families with an autistic association are exposed to the same environmental elements including environmental toxins, foods and people associations as families without autism, the answer could possibly be found outside the genetic link.

Of interest, studies using imaging techniques have identified that children with autism have brains that are slightly larger than those children of the general population who do not have autism. The theory here is that these slightly enlarged brains could be in some way wired differently. This hypothesis is currently under investigation by the University of Pittsburgh.

Another theory being investigated is that there is some problem as yet unidentified in the actions of the body's immune system. However, the National Institute of Health (NIH) has stated that to date the evidence is not strong enough to show a causal relationship. In some ways, if there is a problem with the immune system, then this could be linked back to the genetic theory. The reason being, that genetic links affect the immune system which then has the potential to link back to measles and immunization. A baby's body is unable to effectively deal with an allergy associated with the immunization and this could result in neurological problems.

Moving on to food, some studies have identified that having allergies to certain foods especially gluten which is found in oats, wheat, barley and rye and casein in dairy products may be a contributory factor.

In conclusion, to date no one theory stands out from the rest as being the true cause of autism. Researchers continue to study possible causes and to pin down a definitive answer. Once the cause has been identified, then treatment protocols can be developed to either treat or prevent the syndrome.

3. Symptoms

Autism is a condition that starts in childhood—and it is a condition that you will have for the rest of your life. Affected children usually have problems in three areas of development. These areas are: social skills, language skills and behavior.

It is important to bear in mind, that even though two children may have the same diagnosis, they may act very differently and display very different skills and abilities. In the majority of cases, children with the most severe autism will have a complete inability to speak or interact with other people.

The majority of children will display signs of autism in their early infant months. However, there have been case studies where children appeared to be developing normally for the first few months or possibly the first year or two of life, then, for some reason they suddenly became withdrawn or lose skills that they have already acquired.

In some of these cases a common trigger may be the cause. The research has not yet proven that these triggers are responsible for the deterioration in development levels of these children.

In fact each child will have their own plan of development. However, there are common signs which determine the symptoms of an autistic disorder.

A child with autism may fail to respond to their name, exhibit poor eye contact with others, may appear not to hear at all on some occasions; they may also resist cuddling and holding; in addition, they may appear unaware of the feelings of others towards them and they may be classified as loners as they prefer to play by themselves.

The second category that affects a child with autism is their language development. A child with autism will start talking at a later stage in their life than other children. In addition, they may lose the ability to express previously learnt words or sentences.

Children who have autism will rarely make eye contact with others and they will often use a different rhythm or tone when they do speak. As an example, their speech can appear mechanical or a sing-song type.

Parents of children with autism will often find that their children find it difficult to commence a conversation, or to keep the conversation moving along. They will often repeat words or phrases verbatim but will find it extremely difficult to know in what context to use the words themselves.

In the third development category parents will often find that their children's behavior will develop differently to other children. As an example, they may perform repetitive movements such as rocking backwards and forwards or spinning, or they may prefer to perform a repetitive action such as hand flapping.

These children will develop routines that they feel comfortable with, and will often become agitated at any changes to their routine. Children with autism rarely stay still—they prefer constant movement.

They are often drawn to moving objects such as spinning wheels on a toy car, they can also be ultra-sensitive to bright lights, sounds and to touch; however, they appear to be oblivious to actions or situations that may cause pain in other people.

A child with autism will usually have trouble explaining a situation to others. As an example, when a parent reads a book to a child who does not have autism, they will often point to pictures and have a running commentary with their parents about the contents of the book. By comparison, a child with autism will rarely point at pictures and will not start a dialogue concerning the contents of the book. Being able to interact in this way at an early age is an important early learning ability that is needed as a child grows up and develops their language and social skills.

As a child with autism grows up they will become more withdrawn from other people, in comparison to a child who does not suffer from autism who will become more engaged with others and develop many friendships.

Children with autism will also experience more learning difficulties and will also have difficulty acquiring useful skills, more so than children who do not have autism. Generally, children with autism will often have a normal range of intelligence when compared to those who have IQs lower than normal. Interestingly, some children with autism will grow up to have an exceptional skill in such endeavors as music, math or electronics.

4. Diagnosis

A definitive diagnosis of autism is usually made when a child reaches the age of three or four. In order to confirm the diagnosis, a specific number of criteria have to be met as defined in the diagnostic and statistical manual of mental disorders—IV (DSM-IV). The reason that physicians like to make a diagnosis at age three or four is because the general range of normal behavior is so extensive that there is a possibility a child could simply be a slow developer.

In my own particular case, I was a very slow developer. And I do not have autism or any other neurological or behavioral problems. In fact, I did not really get my act together until I was 15 years old. After then, I seemed to really catch up with a rush.

At university I got a degree in economics, accountancy and business administration, although I never pursued a career in those fields. Instead, I decided to concentrate on natural health research—something I have done for the past 37 years.

Parents are often the best judge of their child's behavior and if they feel that their child is different in any way, and they suspect that autism or some other disorder may be involved, then they should consult their physician about their concerns, expressing reasons why they believe that their child is not developing normally.

Being diagnosed with autism is a serious business that will last a lifetime. This is why an early diagnosis can result in many of the behaviors associated with autism being positively treated, to a level whereby, the sufferer would appear normal to an untrained eye. However, adults and children who are older, who have more severe autism, may portray odd behavior which has the effect of making it difficult for them to make friends. On the plus side, they will often be able to live independent lives and be able to pursue a career.

At the baby stage, there are various things that parents can watch out for that may identify potential problems in the months ahead. One of these is, does a baby responding to their name? Of interest, videotaped studies viewed in later years have shown that children with autism usually only respond to their name approximately 20 percent of the time. However it is important to bear in mind that a lack of response to their name, or other sounds, could indicate that the child may have a hearing deficiency.

Further criteria may be to do with the parents more than the child. If the parents portray limited facial expressions or behavior patterns than this can have an effect on the child. Studies show that an infant who is as young as 8 to 10 months will imitate clapping, facial expressions and laughing with their parents. This is a normal bonding action between a child and its parents. Many infant games are involved here, such as peek-a-boo and patty cake, patty cake bakers man. It is worth noting, that children with autism will have less interaction with their parents than children who do not have autism.

Another indicator could be if the baby responds socially to others. At a very early age children will respond to others by smiling and gurgling. As an example when a baby hears another baby cry they may start to cry themselves, or look worried. A baby who is a little older may crawl over to the baby who is upset and try and comfort them. Researchers as well as parents have observed that children with autism do not do this. For some reason they seem oblivious to the emotions and feelings of others.

An infant who is developing normally will want to engage their parent in what they are doing; for example, drawing the parent's attention to a toy they are playing with or pointing at different objects. This engagement process usually begins at around age one.

A casual observer may notice that the baby watches the parent and then identifies what the parent is watching. This watching sequence is lacking in children with autism. For some reason these children are totally unaware of the interest shown by the parent in what they are doing. They rarely ever show their toys to their parents.

Other indicators may include the baby not displaying purposeful gestures by the time they are one years old, additionally they don't speak at all by the age of 16 months and additionally they have poor eye contact with their parents. Another indicator is that they have difficulty in knowing how to play with their toys, or they often become attached to just one object and rarely if ever smile. On occasions these children seem to have hearing difficulties as a result of only projecting selective hearing.

The process of reaching a definitive conclusion regarding whether a child has autism or not can be time-consuming. The American Academy of Neurology state that it can be two to three years after a child's parent's first notice that something is wrong before a diagnosis is made. Physicians are ever mindful of not labeling a child as having autism when some other condition could be causing the problem.

It can be a fine line between diagnosing a child who may or may not have autism. By making a correct diagnosis, treatment protocols can be implemented that could help to reverse some of the behavior patterns that have the potential to create such a negative impact on a child's life.

Parents who are concerned that their child could have autism or some other disorder should not of necessity wait for a definitive diagnosis to be made before treatment commences. Some treatments that can be investigated include physical therapy, speech therapy and occupational therapy. These early-stage treatments will not restrict the progression of a typical infant, and will in fact have a positive benefit on a child with autism.

Regarding insurance companies, to get these therapies paid for will only require a diagnosis concerning developmental delay without the classification that the child has autism.

A recent study published on June 26, 2012 in the online open access Journal BMC medicine, featured a new test developed by researchers at Boston Children's Hospital. This uses a technique called electroencephalogram (EEG) which involves placing 24 electrodes on a child's scalp.

This test helped them identify 33 patterns that connect brain regions which were different in 430 children with autism whose ages ranged between two and 12. This compared with 554 neurotypical controls.

Should the test be validated, then it will be a quicker and simpler way of determining a diagnosis of autism. This new test is very simple to perform because the electrodes can be put in place on the scalp in a few minutes, as they come prefabricated into a head net. Patients can move around if they wish while wearing the net, and the big plus, the readings only take approximately 20 minutes to complete.

This new test could provide a more accurate and reliable way of determining a diagnosis of autism than is done at present, whereby the diagnosis is determined by observing a child's behavior and assessing their clinical history.

For parents, it is important for them to continue to ask questions that satisfy their concerns regarding their child. Being well informed and discussing treatment options will enable them to move forward. It is advisable not to wait for a definitive diagnosis in order to start the treatment process. By commencing an early intervention this will give the child the best possible chance to get over many of the hurdles which result from their autistic condition.

5. Different Types of Autism

There are five types of developmental brain disorders that are commonly known as Autism Spectrum Disorders. These are briefly described as follows:

Autism:

Children diagnosed with this condition find it difficult to interact with others. The outside world may appear intimidating to such people and as a consequence, will react accordingly. Children with this condition may perform repetitive behavior. Their interaction with others may prove difficult for them as they have difficulty performing verbally and nonverbally.

Childhood Disintegrative Disorder:

This condition is characterized by the child having not only the loss of verbal communication, but also bladder and bowel issues as well. This condition affects males and females equally. This is a rare condition. In general, symptoms will normally appear in a child between the age of two and four years, and until that age development will be normal.

Rett Syndrome:

This disorder usually appears after a period of normal development between the ages of six and 18 months. Following this period of normal development, the child changes socially and mentally. This is a rare condition which usually affects females only. As in other autistic conditions, there is difficulty with verbal communication as well as social skills. In addition, repetitive behavior patterns are also abnormal.

Pervasive Developmental Disorder:

Symptoms of this condition usually appear before the age of three years, and is best represented by difficulties in verbal communication and social interaction. This is a one-size-fits-all category for children who have signs or symptoms that are common in one category. In addition, they also display symptoms from other categories as well.

Asperger Syndrome:

This is a disorder that affects development in both verbal communication and social skill areas. This is best described as a child who is totally focused on one particular topic and is only interested in all aspects of that topic. They often become experts in their particular topic and develop an educated speech pattern to describe it. In all probability they will experience difficulty with interaction on mundane routines that they will need to carry out. Additionally, they will also have problems with their nonverbal skills and in many cases will exhibit uncoordinated movements.

Treatments for the above conditions may or may not include medication, but therapy will definitely be involved. This therapy should include modification of behavior, socialization as well as verbal and nonverbal communication skills, in order to assist the child in coping with their condition.

If you suspect that your child is displaying any of the signs and symptoms described above then you should discuss this with your child's pediatrician so that an assessment may be undertaken, and an appropriate treatment plan can be put in place. For a child to gain maximum benefit from a treatment plan, it is best if it is commenced as soon as possible.

6. Risk Factors

Various risk factors have been identified as being a potential cause of developing autism. Knowing these risk factors gives researchers a way to better understand how research should be directed to finally discover both causes and cures for the condition. Areas that are currently under investigation include: the mother's general health during pregnancy, exposure to viruses during pregnancy, delivery problems and other environmental factors.

Current estimates have determined that roughly between three to six children out of every thousand will develop autism. Boys are four times more likely to develop autism than girls; but when girls develop autism the condition is more likely to be severe. The condition does appear to run in families, however, the condition is not contagious. Of interest, twins are extremely likely to share the condition, and identical twins in most cases will both develop autism.

Research has identified that children who have food allergies, digestive disorders, seizures, disturbed sleep patterns, bipolar disorders, obsessions, compulsive disorders, and sensory disorders demonstrate a higher risk of developing autism than children who do not have these conditions.

Aluminum and Autism

Aluminum is widely used in food packaging, and is often included in many household products. You'll find it in antacids, toothpaste tubes, deodorants, aluminum foil, cooking utensils, as well as water that you drink.

Fortunately, only in certain circumstances will aluminum enter the body. If old aluminum cookware is used to heat an acidic element such as: tea, tomatoes or rhubarb then aluminum particles will be leached into the water. In addition, if you are deficient in zinc, then you will tend to absorb more aluminum.

Of particular concern aluminum, like many other toxic metals binds itself to essential vitamins and minerals, thereby making these essential nutrients unavailable to the body.

It is well known that aluminum toxicity is implicated in a loss of brain function and memory. Aluminum has also been linked to kidney difficulties in babies as well as behavioral problems and autism in older children.

The Age of the Child

The age of the child is also a risk factor for developing autism. A child who is under three years of age has a higher risk of developing the condition than a child who is older than three years of age. Additionally, children who have relatively rare genetic disorders, for example: tuberous sclerosis, fragile X. syndrome, neurofibromatosis, phenylketonuria (PKU) or epilepsy, are also at higher risk of developing the condition.

Environmental and Genetic Factors

A significant five year study which commenced in November 2007 by researchers from Kaiser Permanente and the California Department of Public Health, in addition to five other sites around the US, are investigating environmental and genetic factors that may cause autism. The study criterion is set to involve 2,700 children and their families from six different areas of the United States who were born between September 2003 and August 2005. Areas that will be studied include: environmental factors, socio demographic information, genetics and family medical history.

Schizophrenia and Autism May Be Linked in Families

New research from Sweden and Israel which was published on July 6, 2012 in the Journal of psychiatry suggests that in families where there is a history of schizophrenia or bipolar disorder then they are more likely to have a child with autism.

In particular, where parents have been diagnosed with schizophrenia their children were nearly three times as likely to have autism and/or Asperger syndrome. With regard to bipolar disorder, the link was weaker, but still consistent.

The researchers theorized that there could be certain gene mutations that are passed from parent to child.

The number of children being diagnosed with autism in the United States is rising steadily according to the Centers for Disease Control and Prevention (CDC). They estimate that one in 88 children has an autism spectrum disorder. That is an increase from one in 150 just 10 years ago.

For this new study, researchers evaluated data from three separate databases. Two of these related to children and families in Sweden, together with their medical diagnosis, and a third related to Israeli citizens who were entering the army draft, including sibling pairs. In total the research team had data on over 30,000 young people who have autism.

The researchers discovered that the children from Sweden whose parents or a sibling had been diagnosed with schizophrenia were 2.6 to 2.9 times more likely to have autism. The same figures related to the Israeli study group.

The general consensus is that while two things may share a risk factor, this does not mean that they are the same thing. Concerning the needs of people with autism and schizophrenia, and the treatments that are available that are known to work for one condition or the other, it is known for a fact that they do not overlap very well.

7. Treatments

Various treatments are available for children with autism that appear to have a positive effect on their actions and reactions. The common aim of these treatments is to improve a child's social skills and behavior and language abilities, a common goal being that they will be able to function independently.

Children who have only mild symptoms of autism are often capable of functioning well in adulthood. On the other hand, children whose symptoms are more severe will have a greater challenge as they go through life.

There are many treatments available and I have described a few of them in this book. However, you may wish to do some research yourself, possibly using the Internet, as there is a lot of information available for you to digest. But please be mindful that a lot of information put on the Internet is purely speculative, and some of it has very little validity.

Briefly, treatment protocols fall into various categories as follows: treatments that are approved by a government body, treatments where some research is currently in progress, alternative treatments, treatments that are backed by sound case studies and finally, treatments that may be described as being at the cutting edge where there is currently no available data.

Whatever path you choose to follow, the main criteria should be the child's welfare, and no treatments plan that you decide to follow should have a negative impact on a child's development.

Drug Treatments

Let me start with drug treatments. These are quite common, however, they won't cure the condition but they may assist in managing behavioral conditions. In addition, they may also help to manage depression and/or seizures. I have included some commonly prescribed medications in the next chapter.

Of interest, there is some evidence to suggest that an overgrowth of candida albicans— a yeast which may release toxins into the system. This can cause autistic symptoms as well as damage to the central nervous system, in addition to the immune system.

Autism related to an allergy condition will usually show up in the first three years of a child's life, but not necessarily as an infant. There is a theory that allergies will have a negative impact on the immune system which will then trigger the nervous system to perform abnormally.

Auditory Training

In addition to music therapy auditory training is often used to help improve the language development skills of children. Research has shown that children with autism often have sensory dysfunction. Auditory training helps stimulate sensory functions of the brain.

The Delacato Method

This method is often used with children who have suffered brain injuries as a result of an accident. It is used for cross patterning, as well as patterning and sensory exercises to help improve memory processing. In addition, this treatment is also being used with autistic children to help the brain improve nerve connections.

The Lovaas Method

This method has been practiced for over 30 years and is basically a program designed to modify behavior patterns. The downside of this method is that it needs a fully trained person to work with a child for roughly 40 hours each week.

Picture Exchange Communication System

This is a method that was developed for children who have nonverbal communication difficulties. It is designed to help a child communicate better from a nonverbal standpoint.

TEACCH

To give it its full name: Treatment and Education of Autistic and Related Communication Handicapped Children. It is basically a management program designed to deliver more balanced behavior in autistic children.

In this program speech and occupational therapy are activated to assist children to develop their language skills, and fine motor (nerve) skills, by using a home study program given to the parents. This program requires a daily one or two hours input by the parents

Vitamin Therapy

Vitamin therapy can also be used. This therapy uses DMG (dimethylglycine) which is a substance obtained from brown rice and liver. The chemical construction of this compound is similar to vitamin B15. You do not require a prescription, and it can be obtained from health food stores. And on the upside, it does not have any side effects. Parents who have used DMG have noticed improvements in speech, eye contact, social behavior skills as well as an improved attention span. Vitamin B6 can be added after approximately two weeks to help counteract any hyperactivity that may have occurred.

To carry vitamin and mineral therapy further, I have included a section on nutritional supplements elsewhere in this book.

Flxyx Therapy

This is a photo simulation technique which is being developed by Dr. Ochs. To date there have been no clinical trials or results of someone using this therapy.

Changes to the Diet

Changes to the diet of an artistic child, especially eliminating gluten which is found in oats, barley, wheat and rye as well as casein which is found in dairy products—especially milk, could have a positive effect. Alternatives could include gluten free grains and flour as well as rice, and for dairy products, soy milk, and tofu or rice milk.

Researchers theorize that these elements are somehow absorbed differently in the body of an autistic child, and as a result, provide a false sensory reading in the brain. This particular condition is not linked to an allergic response—such as celiac disease or being lactose intolerant. Currently studies are on-going to better understand this phenomenon in a number of centers.

It is important to discuss any changes to your child's diet with your child's health care provider before you commence.

8. Medications

No medication is available, that has been proven to address the main characteristics that children with autism show, in such things as communication skills and social relationships. However, for some children, medication can relieve behavioral situations which are linked to autism.

Making a decision to try medication on your child can be a difficult one. The important thing is to weigh up the possible benefits against the possible side effects.

Medication is often considered where there are situations that the child may self-harm, or where there are other severe characteristics which are not responding to other treatments.

Medications for a child with autism are usually prescribed by a pediatrician or a child and adolescent psychiatrist. If you decide to choose a doctor to prescribe medications for your child, then make sure this person has experience in working with children with autism.

Medications and Possible Side Effects

As mentioned above, it is important to weigh up the benefits, versus the possible side effects of any medication that you propose having prescribed for your child. The following are some of the medications and their known side effects which are commonly prescribed for children with autism, although many of these medications will be prescribed for other conditions as well.

Children with Hyperactive Behavior

Stimulant drugs which are used to treat attention-deficit/hyperactivity disorder (ADHD) may also help some individuals with autism. The reason being, these drugs help a person to concentrate and focus their attention in addition to reducing their impulsive nature and tendency to be hyperactive.

Methylphenidate (Ritalin, Concerta)

Warning! You have to be careful how you use this medication, especially if there are issues with emotional problems, or alcohol or substance abuse. If abuse is an issue, then the medication may not be as effective. In addition, any abuse involving this medication may lead to addiction and severe mental reorientation. If taking the medication is suddenly stopped, then, the patient may suffer from depression and other mental problems. If a decision is made to no longer take this medication, then a doctor should slowly reduce the dose over a period of time.

In the US there are over 8 million children being prescribed Ritalin. What is alarming is that this habit forming amphetamine has many similar properties to cocaine.

Methylphenidate

This is a central nervous system stimulant, it is not known however, how it accomplishes this.

Methylphenidate

This is primarily a treatment for attention deficit disorder (ADD). In addition, it is also prescribed for uncontrollable periods of daytime sleep (narcolepsy).

Available research and testing has identified that these medications can reduce hyperactive behavior in children who have autism. The benefits of this medication might enable children to focus on a specific task for longer period of time, and give more thought to a particular subject before they act.

Dexmethylphenidate (Focalin)

Dexmethylphenidate is primarily a treatment for attention deficit disorder (ADD). It may also be prescribed for other conditions as well.

It is also a central nervous system stimulant, it is not known however, how it accomplishes this.

Amphetamine

Amphetamine is primarily a stimulant and an appetite suppressant. It stimulates the nerves and brain which make up part of the central nervous system. It achieves this by elevating specific body chemicals. This has the effect of increasing blood pressure as well as heart rate, and at the same time—reduces appetite.

This medication is prescribed as a treatment for narcolepsy—a sleep disorder in addition to attention deficit disorder with hyperactivity (ADHD).

In addition, this medication may be prescribed for other conditions as directed by a doctor.

Dextroamphetamine (Dexedrine)

Warning! This medication may become habit-forming if used over a long period of time. It is important to use this medication only as prescribed by a doctor. It is also important, not to share this medication with other people. If this medication is abused, then it can cause serious heart problems, blood vessel problems, or in extreme cases, death.

Dextroamphetamine is a stimulant for the central nervous system. It is not known how it accomplishes this. It assists in the improvement of attention span and behavior by affecting certain brain chemicals.

This medication is used for children who have hyperactivity and attention deficit disorders. It is also prescribed to treat narcolepsy—a sleep disorder. In addition, it may also be prescribed for other conditions.

Lisdexamfetamine (Vyvanase)

Warning! The same warning applies as mentioned for Dextroamphetamine (Dexedrine).

Lisdexamfetamine is an amphetamine. Therefore it is a stimulant for the central nervous system. It is not known how it accomplishes this. It assists in the improvement of attention span and behavior by affecting certain brain chemicals.

This medication is prescribed for attention deficit hyperactivity disorder (ADHD) and is incorporated as part of a total treatment program. This program could include psychological, educational, and social components. In addition, it may also be prescribed for other conditions as decided by a doctor.

Common side effects for the medications in this section include:

A lowering of appetite is the main side effect of these medications. The downside of this side effect could mean that a child might lose weight, or possibly not gain weight. Another issue if their appetite is reduced, then they will be less likely to get sufficient nutrients in the form of vitamins and minerals to help nourish their bodies. This could exacerbate the building of neurons in the brain which are needed for various motor functions of the body, as well as memory function.

Additional side effects may include:

- Jerky body movements
- An increase in repetitive behavior
- An increased level of anxiety
- An increased level of hyperactive behavior

Children with Obsessive Behavior and Anxiety Issues

Selective Serotonin Reuptake Inhibitors (SSRIs) are a class of antidepressants that are often prescribed to lower anxiety and treat conditions of obsessive compulsive disorder (OCD), which are often observed in children with autism.

Citalopram (Celexa)

Citalopram (Celexa) works by restoring the balance of the neurotransmitter serotonin which is a natural substance in the brain. This medication helps to improve mood.

Escitalopram (Lexapro)

Escitalopram influences brain chemicals that could possibly become unstable and cause symptoms of depression or anxiety.

This medication is prescribed as a treatment for anxiety in adults, in addition to major depressive disorders in adults and adolescents who have attained the minimum of 12 years of age.

Fluoxetine (Prozac, Prozac Weekly, Rapiflux, Sarafem, Selfemra)

Fluoxetine works by restoring the balance of the neurotransmitter serotonin which is a natural substance in the brain. This medication helps to improve mood.

When these brain chemicals become unbalanced, this can cause depression, panic, anxiety, or obsessive compulsive symptoms.

In addition, Fluoxetine may on occasions be combined with another medication called olanzapine (Zyprexa). This combination is used to treat depression caused by bipolar disorder (manic depression).

Another use for this combination is to treat cases of depression following the prescribing of at least two other medications which have proved unsuccessful.

Fluvoxamine (Luvox)

Fluvoxamine (Luvox) influences brain chemicals that could possibly become unstable and cause symptoms of obsessive-compulsive disorder.

This medication is prescribed to treat cases of social anxiety disorder (social phobia), or obsessive-compulsive disorders which involve repeated thoughts or actions.

Paroxetine (Paxil)

Paroxetine (Paxil) works by restoring the balance of the neurotransmitter serotonin which is a natural substance in the brain. This medication helps to improve mood.

This medication is prescribed for cases of depression or obsessive compulsive disorder (OCD). In addition, it may be prescribed to treat panic disorders or post-traumatic stress disorder (PTSD). Other uses for this medication include: social anxiety disorder and general anxiety disorder.

Sertraline (Zoloft)

Sertraline influences brain chemicals that could possibly become unstable and cause depression, panic, anxiety, or symptoms of obsessive-compulsive disorder.

This medication is prescribed for cases of post-traumatic stress disorder (PTSD), in addition to premenstrual dysphoric disorder (PMDD).

Common side effects of SSRIs include:

- Stomach problems (stomach pain and feelings of sickness)
- Difficulty sleeping
- Irritability and nervous conditions

Teenagers as well as grown-ups can have sexual dysfunction when taking SSRIs

A worrying trend: scientists are concerned that people taking SSRIs may consider hurting themselves or even committing suicide, especially if they are less than 25 years of age. Should these feelings happen, it is nearly always within the first two weeks of starting a medication, therefore a careful watch should be kept on the patient during this period.

Children with Jerky Movements

Children with autism frequently have jerky movements these could also be referred to as repetitive movements, which children seem unable to control. These movements frequently happen in children's shoulders or facial area. On occasions, children will also frequently clear their throats or make grunting sounds.

With some children these jerky movements occur frequently and as a result, make the child feel uncomfortable. If this is a problem with your child, then you may need to consider a medication approach.

Various medications can be prescribed to help control repetitive movements. These medications include antipsychotics such as Clonidine. Clonidine can also assist in lowering hyperactivity behavior.

Common side effects of antipsychotics include:

- Weight gain
- Drooling
- Sleepiness and a feeling of tiredness

Clonidine

Has the effect of making children feel very sleepy. Some children can also experience a drop in blood pressure or heart rate. It can be especially dangerous if too much of this medication is taken, therefore it should be stored out of reach of children.

Children with Aggressive behavior

One of the symptoms of autism is that children can become very aggressive towards other people. In addition, on occasions they can break or damage things. Additionally, some children also self-harm by beating their head against a solid object.

Antipsychotic drugs are often prescribed for this condition.

Risperidone (Risperdal)

Risperdal is an antipsychotic medication. It is an "atypical antipsychotic". Its main effect is to change the actions of various chemicals in the brain.

Risperdal is often used to treat schizophrenia and bipolar disorder (manic depression). In addition, it is also prescribed for autistic children who have symptoms of irritability.

Risperidone (Risperdal) has been approved by the Food and Drug Administration (FDA) as a treatment for irritability, aggression, and self-harming actions in children and adolescents who have autism.

Olanzapine (Zyprexa)

Olanzapine is an antipsychotic medication. Its main effect is to change the actions of various chemicals in the brain.

Olanzapine is often used to treat psychotic conditions such as schizophrenia and bipolar disorder (manic depression) in adults and children who have a minimum age of at least 13 years.

Olanzapine is occasionally prescribed together with other antipsychotic or antidepressant medications.

Abilify (Aripiprazole)

Abilify (aripiprazole) is classed as an antipsychotic medication. Its main effect is to change the actions of various chemicals in the brain.

In addition, Abilify is often used for the treatment of irritability, aggression, mood swings, temper tantrums, and self-injury as a result of an autistic disorder in children who are at least six years old.

Abilify (Aripiprazole) has been approved by the Food and Drug Administration (FDA) as a treatment for irritability, aggression, and self-harming actions in children and adolescents who have autism.

Quetiapine (Seroquel)

Quetiapine (Seroquel) is classed as an antipsychotic medicine. Its main effect is to change the actions of various chemicals in the brain.

It is used to treat schizophrenia in adults as well as children who have reached a minimum age of 13 years.

Quetiapine is used to treat bipolar disorder (manic depression) in adults as well as children who have reached a minimum age of 10 years.

In addition, Quetiapine is often used together with antidepressant medications for major depressive disorders in adults.

Extended-release quetiapine (Seroquel XR) should only be prescribed for adults and should not be prescribed for anyone younger than 18 years of age.

Common side effects of atypical antipsychotics include:

- Weight gain

- Drooling

- Feelings of tiredness or sleepiness

Additional side effects may include:

- Uncontrollable jerky movements, in addition to stiff arms or legs

- Metabolic changes in the hormone prolactin, this can cause milk secretion as well as breast development

- Serious changes in how the body controls blood sugar levels, the quantity of fats in the body, and the liver. All these are of prime concern to children's well-being.

Children with Sleeping Difficulties

Quite a few children with autism often wake up during the night or have trouble sleeping. The hormone melatonin which is synthesized in the pineal gland—a small gland in the brain, is responsible for making a person sleep. Melatonin can be obtained as a supplement from health food stores. In addition, various amounts of melatonin are also found in many fruits and vegetables such as: grape skins, tomatoes, tart cherries and walnuts.

One of the possible side effects of taking melatonin is that a child may feel sick or get a headache, especially if they've been taking it for some time. Some adults claim that they have an "out of sorts" feeling the following day after taking melatonin.

Seizures

Approximately one third of people with autism experience seizures at some time during their lives—some people experience many seizures.

Anti-epilepsy medications are often used to treat this condition effectively. There are quite a few anti-epilepsy medications, therefore the most effective one will depend on the type of seizure. In addition, which one will be prescribed will depend on what other medications the child may be taking.

Common side effects of medications prescribed for seizures include:

- Feelings of sleepiness
- Changes in behavior
- Stomach problems

How to Assess if a Medication is Working

Your child will need to be monitored carefully by yourself and your doctor when they start taking a new medication.

You need to consider what particular condition your child is taking the medication for before they commence. Then over the following week or weeks write down details of when and how often the condition occurs, also write down the severity of the condition. Also observe your child's sleeping habits and whether there have been any changes in the appetite. By writing everything down, you'll be able to gain a reasonable understanding of whether the medication is working or not.

It is also important not to make any changes concerning their routine or other therapies they may be partaking in. This way, there will be no additional factors which may cause any changes in the child.

Additionally you may ask a family member or friend—someone who is not aware that your child has started taking a new medication and ask them if they have noticed any changes in your child's behavior. If this other person observes a positive change in your child's behavior then this is a good indication that the medication is working.

Additional Things to Consider and Discuss with your Healthcare Provider

Each child with autism is different, and each one has different needs. Therefore, a few different medications and dosage levels may have to be tried to find the most effective one.

Frequently a medication may need to be taken in a specific way for it to be most effective. It is best therefore to talk to your child's doctor about when and how often your child needs to take their medication, also whether it should be taken with or without food.

It is important not to suddenly stop taking a medication, especially if your child has been taking it for a long period of time. It is best to talk to your child's doctor if you are considering whether your child should stop taking a particular medication.

As most medications were originally designed for adults, the effects they may have on children may not always be known.

9. Clinical Trials

There are currently many clinical trials underway to treat autism and find more effective treatment protocols. The purpose of many of these trials is to find new ways to improve overall patient care and at the same time, improve patient health.

Trials are conducted to see whether new drugs are going to be safe and effective for use, in addition to new procedures and devices that may in the future become effective treatment options.

In the case of autism, these trials are conducted as a means to answer scientific questions, as well as the other purposes described above. Some of these trials may be open to new volunteers and if you are interested, it is best to register your interest with your doctor and/or enquire through a university or hospital.

One purpose of any clinical trial is to determine if there are any unacceptable risks and side effects. The risks and side effects will be categorized as either mild which may cause only a small amount of discomfort or inconvenience, or something that could be more severe and possibly life-threatening.

In each individual trial the risks and benefits will be carefully weighed. The majority of clinical trials are divided into different phases that are designed to focus on determining an answer to a particular scientific research question.

Here are the different phases of a clinical trial.

phase 1. This often comprises a very small group of participants. The purpose of this phase is to evaluate the safety of a particular drug and what a safe dosage would be. In addition, any specific side effects will be noted and evaluated. This phase could also involve a new procedure to determine whether it will be effective or not.

Phase 2. If phase 1 is successful, the trial will be repeated using a larger group of participants, using the same parameters as in phase 1.

Phase 3. In the third phase an even larger group of participants will be used, but this time a comparison will be made with conventional treatments that are already in use to determine overall effectiveness and safety.

Phase 4. The last phase will monitor long-term effects of a treatment after it has become available.

Here is one example of a clinical study that was conducted regarding autism. There was much speculation whether the hormone secretin could be a treatment option for autism. Dr. Katrina Williams at the Children's Hospital, Westmeade, Australia did an evaluation of the results from 14 different studies concerning whether secretin would prove beneficial for treating and controlling autism. She determined following various tests that secretin was not suitable as a treatment option.

The above example is just one of many clinical studies that are currently being conducted to find an effective treatment for autism. These trials are important for finding effective treatment options, and having the help of volunteers, who take part in these studies, is critical in finding different ways to reduce the effects of this disorder. You can find out what clinical trials are currently taking place by going to http://clinicaltrials.gov/. This is a really useful site.

10. Dietary Guidelines.

Certain evidence supports the link between food additives and preservatives which has an impact on mental ability. If your child appears to have food sensitivities, then this should be investigated. Certain foods can be termed as sensitive, these include dairy products, nuts, grains containing gluten (oats, wheat, barley, rye), and eggs.

It is also important to incorporate high fiber content into the diet. This should include such things as raw fruits, vegetables, whole grains, cereals with a high fiber content per serving and legumes. In addition, lean meat will be beneficial, as well as oily fish such as salmon, tuna, mackerel, and sardines.

One of the problems with the average diet today, is that a lot of essential nutrients—and especially minerals, are no longer present in the soil due to excessive farming techniques. Another issue is the use of pesticides and other chemicals that are sprayed onto the land to kill bugs and enhance crop growing times.

Cattle and poultry are often injected with antibiotics and growth hormones in an intensive farming environment to bring the end product that much quicker to the consumer.

Therefore, it is essential wherever possible and practical to purchase organic produce whether it is fruit, vegetables, meat or poultry. It is also, as mentioned above, important to incorporate oily fish into the diet.

It is best to avoid white sugar, drinks containing caffeine such as coffee and cola, processed foods that contain high levels of nitrates, sodium, artificial colors, and other preservatives.

It will be beneficial to keep blood sugar at a normal level by preparing several small meals each day rather than one or two large ones.

Get Your Kids off to a Good Start

Starting your children off with good dietary habits will benefit them for the rest of their lives. This is probably the greatest contribution you can make to their overall development. Sadly, today, we have a snack culture whereby everyone is bombarded with advertisements for junk food, and every time you go into the supermarket, there is an abundance of easy to cook ready meals with enticing pictures of the ready meal on the packaging. It is no wonder that there is a great temptation to go down this route.

It can therefore be difficult to get your children into good eating habits, especially if their peers are going down the junk food route. But the effort you put in will be well worth it in the years ahead.

How to Develop Good Eating Habits

It is interesting how the body craves things that are not go for it. Take sugar as an example. This is an acquired taste through eating sweet foods. This tendency can be overcome by gradually reducing the sweetness in foods and drinks. One of the best ways to achieve this is to substitute sweetened drinks with fruit juice.

Most children don't drink enough water. Try and avoid water from the faucet if at all possible. In many areas of the country, water supplied by the public utility is full of chemicals. Fluoride which is a waste by-product of aluminum production is often added. Therefore, it is best to drink either bottled water, or water that has been through a filtration system.

If at all possible, try and avoid offering sweetened foods, cola and any other sweetened drinks and candies. If you do, then psychology kicks in here, and these types of foods and drinks will have been associated with something good that has happened. This kind of association can then carry on through life, which can have health consequences later on.

Cola type drinks are very high in sugar and caffeine. Caffeine is an addictive drug. What I find amazing is that you have to reach a certain age in order to smoke or consume alcohol, yet, a very young child can buy a cola drink which is high in an addictive substance, with all the subsequent health problems that this can entail.

Let us now look at breakfast cereals. Very few of these are sugar free. There is an insidious thing going on here, whereby food manufacturers assist children to develop a craving for something sweet at a very early age. Most cereal products contain fast releasing sugars, and often have additional sugar added. Many of these cereal products are also very low in fiber—but the packaging looks good!

Try and purchase unsweetened whole-grain cereals and encourage your children to sweeten their cereals with fruit such as sliced banana, apple, pear, raspberries or blueberries.

Berry fruits make excellent snacks. It is therefore a good idea to always have these available for your children to snack on. Try and send them off to school with a piece of fruit.

As your children get older, there is always a tendency for them to copy their peers, and this will in all probability start by eating sweet things. However, if during their early years they are being discouraged from consuming sweetened foods and drinks then they are less likely to acquire an addiction as they get older.

Try developing in your children the habit of eating vegetables, and especially raw ones with each meal. Many times children see vegetables as the best way to ruin their day, so somehow try and figure out a way to make vegetables look enticing. One of the problems with vegetables is that they are often cooked to destruction and as a result do not taste good.

Try and purchase organic vegetables as much as possible. They will not have been sprayed with pesticides or other chemicals. They will be better for you, and will taste good too. Raw organic carrots, peas, parsnip chips—which can be made by steam frying them in diluted soy sauce, as well as mashed and baked potatoes are naturally quite sweet and are often a favorite with children.

Finally desserts. Try and think of healthy desserts—something that is not full of sugar. I find that desserts are an acquired taste. And once that taste is established, it seems to last a lifetime. On many occasions desserts are full of empty calories, which are not always a good idea, if you're trying to lose weight, or maintain an ideal weight.

Watch for Food Allergies

Many children often have a bad reaction to food additives, such as dairy products, peanuts, gluten in grains, household detergents, house dust mites and vehicle exhaust fumes. Some children have an allergic reaction to oranges and eggs. You can watch out for the tell-tale signs of a food allergy. Here are a few examples for you to consider:

Digestive System: excess gas, stomach ache, diarrhea and vomiting, colic.

Intestinal System: irritable bowel disease brought on by stress, Crohn's disease.

Respiratory System: asthma, respiratory system infections, coughing, frequent sore throats, swollen tongue, excessive mucus production.

Skin: eczema, itchy skin, rashes, water retention.

Face: black circles around the eyes, puffiness in the face, runny nose, frequent colds and ear ache, tonsillitis.

Mental State: bedwetting, trouble sleeping and an over emotional state, problems with concentration, hyperactivity.

Many of these challenges will subside once the offending item is identified and removed from the diet. One way to identify allergic food items is to remove one food item for a period of say 10 days, and see if the symptoms subside. If they do, then you have found the answer. If not, then reintroduce that food item and move on to the next suspect food and try again.

Children in Crisis

It seems that's learning difficulties, attention deficit disorders, autism and cases of depression are on the increase. With this increase, there seems to be an emphasis on prescribing the medication Ritalin to solve the problem. In the US there are over 8 million children on this medication. What is alarming is that this habit forming amphetamine has many similar properties to cocaine.

Previously autism seemed to occur mainly from birth, or certainly within the first six months of life. However, during the past 10 years there has been a steady increase in what is termed late onset autism which is mainly diagnosed in the second year of life. What is causing this change? Theories suggest that diet, vaccinations, and possibly digestive and intestinal system disorders, including celiac and Crohn's disease may be implicated in some way. However, many of these problems seem to have a connection in some way to the brain.

Brain Health

The brain is an amazing organ, which is about 3 pounds in weight and consists mainly of fat and water; yet it performs some amazing functions. And it all starts when the child is in the fetal stage. It is critical that the fetus receives adequate nutrition at this very early stage, as it will have a profound effect on learning and behavior as a child grows and develops.

Unfortunately many critical nutrients which are essential for brain development such as essential fatty acids and fat soluble vitamins such as vitamin E and the antioxidant mineral zinc are often missing in the average junk food diet. These important nutrients are also essential for proper digestive system health. Unfortunately these essential nutrients are being replaced by foods which are high in sugar, which contain highly processed fats, refined wheat and dairy products.

Foods That Are Toxic

A diet that is high in refined carbohydrates is not a good idea, and especially as many parents think that eating such foods is one of the causes of hyperactivity and aggression in their children. Various studies show that children, who are hyperactive, generally have a higher sugar intake than children who are not hyperactive. It has been found that reducing sugar consumption reduces instances of hyperactivity.

One study of hyperactive children discovered that more than three quarters had an abnormal intolerance to glucose. Glucose is the main fuel for the brain and body, so when blood glucose levels swing violently during the day when the diet comprises mainly refined carbohydrates, stimulants, candy, chocolate, fizzy drinks, with little or no fiber to slow the absorption of glucose, then, it is little wonder that hyperactivity levels as well as concentration and focus will also swing violently as well.

Gluten and Dairy Products

Breast-feeding your child up to the age of at least four months is one way of preventing sensitivity to milk. Milk is also an essential provider of vitamin A, calcium and essential fats.

It has been noted that one of the contributory factors in autism is the by-products of undesirable chemicals from foods that somehow reach the brain via the bloodstream. This is often a consequence of faulty digestion and absorption.

I have mentioned Crohn's disease elsewhere in this book as well as celiac disease. Where these conditions occur, there is often a mal-absorption of essential nutrients, through the small intestine which can affect not only body health, but brain health as well. This has the effect of starving the body of these essential nutrients.

These rogue substances which get into the brain, have the effect of being implicated in many of the behavioral problems found in autistic children.

11. Nutritional Supplements

It is important that all vitamin and mineral supplements are from a natural source—not synthetic. Natural supplements are living elements unlike their synthetic counterparts which are often by-products of chemical formulas. Therefore, it makes sense to take natural supplements which will help to nourish the various body systems which it is designed for.

Various studies have been conducted to show the effectiveness of supplementing with vitamins and minerals to enhance IQ and reduce aggressive tendencies. In one study of 16 children with behavioral and learning difficulties, each child had their individual nutrient needs assessed. Half the children were then given supplements, the other half were given a placebo.

Each child attended a special reading course designed to improve each child's reading age by one year. Over the following 22 weeks, teachers monitored the behavior, reading age and IQ of the children. Those children taking the placebo achieved an average increase in IQ of 8.4 points and reading age by 1.1 years. However the group of children taking supplements increased their IQ by 17.9 points and their reading age increased by 1.8 years.

Various studies have been done in different environments where aggressive tendencies are present, and in each case where a vitamin and supplement program was implemented there was a dramatic reduction in instances of aggressive behavior. Once the supplement program was terminated, then the aggressive tendencies tended to return.

The following nutritional supplements will prove beneficial to anyone who is autistic.

Multi-vitamin and multi-mineral supplement

The purpose of a good quality natural vitamin and mineral supplement is to provide insurance against any dietary shortfall in essential vitamins and minerals that are required by the body, for it to perform its many different functions. If these essential nutrients are lacking in the diet, then the body will take them from the supplement; if they are not needed, then it will pass out harmlessly in the urine.

Vitamin B6 with magnesium

Both these nutrients are required for emotional and mental stability. Studies have shown how beneficial these two are for autistic behavior. A lack of vitamins B6 has been implicated in various mental disturbances.

When vitamin B6 was combined with magnesium, dramatic improvement in 60 autistic children were observed in a double-blind trial. For this to work, vitamin B6 must be taken with magnesium and not on its own. The suggested dosage would be: 150 mg of vitamins B6 in three equal divided doses. Add to this, 1,000 mg of magnesium per day.

Vitamin B complex

All the B. vitamins work together; therefore it is beneficial to take a B. complex supplement. If individual B. vitamins are required—for example vitamin B6—then this can be taken along with the B. complex vitamin.

B vitamins are water soluble and are easily excreted from the body during times of stress; therefore an adequate daily intake is required.

All the B. vitamins are essential for normal mental capacity. Individuals with schizophrenia, learning problems and other mental disorders often suffer from a lack of B vitamins.

One particular study demonstrated how the B. vitamins can effectively treat individuals who suffer from schizophrenia, when these individuals did not gain benefits from psychotropic drug treatments. A suggested dosage would be 50 mg with each meal.

Calcium magnesium

These two minerals work together, and are available as combined supplements. Calcium is well known to calm the nervous system and is critical for normal brain function. In a recent study, 165 boys who suffered from mental disturbances and learning disabilities had a magnesium deficiency. Suggested dosage: 1,000 mg per day. Use a chelated variety. Chelation means that the calcium magnesium supplement is bound to specific amino acids which make it more readily available to the body.

Vitamin D may need to be added to this supplement, as it is necessary for calcium magnesium absorption.

Choline

Choline is essential for synthesis of the neurotransmitter acetyl-choline which is critical for memory function. Choline is found in lecithin which is derived from soy bean extraction. Choline is therefore critical for boosting brain circulation and nerve activity in the brain. The recommended dosage is 1,000 mg per day. However, it is best to check with a healthcare provider before commencing taking this supplement.

Co-enzyme Q10

This is not a vitamin and not a mineral. But it is found in every cell in the body. And due to age, lifestyle and medications that may be taken for various medical conditions, it gets depleted in the body. It improves circulation, and current research projects are underway to determine if it is beneficial for brain disorders. Take as directed on the bottle.

GABA

Gamma Amino Butyric Acid (GABA) is a neurotransmitter which is formed from the non-essential amino acid glutamic acid. Various studies indicate that GABA can be beneficial in reducing hyperactivity, as well as providing a benefit to children with learning problems. Take a daily amount as recommended on the bottle.

Ginkgo biloba

Ginkgo Biloba is an antioxidant herb which supports the circuiatory system of the body. It is very beneficial for brain related disorders. It is very effective at scavenging free radicals in the brain, and as a result, helps boost oxygenation in the brain tissue. Take as directed on the bottle.

Gotu Kola

Gotu Kola is a member of the parsley family. It is often used with children who have problems staying focused and lack concentration. Take a daily amount as recommended on the bottle.

St. John's Wort

This herb is often used to treat cases of mild to moderate depression, in a natural way. As it has antidepressant properties, and is effective in helping to normalize sleep patterns, it is often recommended in cases of autism.

It is best to check with a health care provider before anyone starts taking St. John's Wort. As this herb has monoamine oxidase (MAO) activity, it may interact with any antidepressant medication which is being taken. Take as directed on the bottle with meals.

Tyrosine

Tyrosine is an essential amino acid which is a precursor for the neurotransmitter serotonin. This is a natural way to raise serotonin levels, which helps with mood improvement and mental outlook. Suggested dose. Take as directed on the bottle, with fruit juice on an empty stomach.

Valerian Root

Valerian is a natural source of plant calcium. It is used with great success in Germany as a treatment for behavioral disorders in children. Take a daily amount as recommended on the bottle.

Vitamin A

Vitamin A also known as retinal can be toxic in high doses, however, its active precursor beta carotene which is converted to vitamin A as it is needed by the body, is not toxic at high doses.

As far as autism is concerned and autistic children in particular, many of these children have a problem with visual perception, and as a result, they do not look straight at a person. This condition is often classified as demonstrating social isolation skills. However, the reason for this is that there are more black and white light receptors, which are called rods, around the edge of the eyes vision field than there are in the middle.

Interestingly, if autistic children are given fish oil which contains vitamin A, then they will start looking straight at a person. To get maximum benefit from vitamin A, the daily requirement may have to be at least double the recommended daily allowance (RDA). Elevated levels of beta carotene may provide extra benefits as well.

Good sources of vitamin A include breast milk, organ meats, milk fat, fish and cod liver oil.

Vitamins C

Vitamins C. with added bioflavonoids is an antioxidant which helps to counteract the effects of free radical damage. As it is water soluble, it is easily depleted from the body during times of stress. Vitamin C is available without the bioflavonoids, but it is more beneficial to obtain a supplement that contains them. Take a daily amount as recommended on the bottle.

Zinc

Zinc is an antioxidant mineral and helps to reduce the effects of free radical damage. Researchers discovered some time ago that a zinc deficiency is often possible in children with learning difficulties.

Where I have mentioned recommended dosages for supplements, these recommendations are for adults, this includes anyone over the age of 18 years. It is important to check with your health care provider if any supplement program you propose implementing is for a child under the age of 12 years.

The Benefits of Vitamin B12

Vitamin B12 also known as Cyanocobalamin can provide substantial benefits for children suffering from autism. Vitamins B12 are necessary to maintain healthy nerve cells as well as red blood cells. It is also necessary for the production of DNA in the billions of cells in the body. As it is the largest vitamin that is known, this makes it more difficult to be assimilated by the body.

As vitamins B12 is such a large molecule, the body has developed a means to help absorb the vitamin into our system. This is achieved by the stomach producing a substance called intrinsic factor which attaches to vitamin B12. This then facilitates the absorption of the B12 vitamin into the end of the small intestine.

Good food sources of vitamin B12 include: milk, poultry, red meat, eggs, fish, yogurt and cheese. Some cereals are fortified with vitamins B12, and there are also supplements that an individual can take if they are not getting enough of this vitamin from their diet.

As vitamin B12 is not found in fruits and vegetables, a child who is a vegetarian may have a significant vitamin B12 deficiency. In these cases, B12 supplementation may be essential.

Researchers have discovered that many autistic children have a vitamin B12 deficiency which it is believed may contribute to the severity of the condition, and as a result, make treatment protocols more problematical. In some cases it can appear that the child is being resistant to the treatment being administered.

There are various reasons why autistic child may be deficient in vitamin B12, these include:

- The child may be a picky eater which can lead to a poor dietary intake of not only vitamin B12 but other vitamins and minerals as well.
- The stomach may produce low quantities of intrinsic factor which can then lead to poor absorption of vitamin B12.
- There could be damage to the nervous system as a result of autoimmune antibodies or neurotoxins which can have the effect of making neurons less receptive to normal B12 intakes.

There can be many reasons why a child may have low levels of vitamin B12. But it is important to discuss this with the child's doctor before commencing any course of treatment, including taking vitamin B12 supplements.

One of the best approaches is to ensure the child is receiving sufficient amounts of vitamin B12 in their diet. If you feel that this is not the case, then it is best to discuss this with your child's doctor to see if supplementing with B12 supplements will prove beneficial.

Essential Fatty Acids and Intelligence

Essential fatty acids which include omega-3 and Omega-6 oils are not made in the body but must be obtained from the diet, and they are critical for many important body functions. Dietary deficiencies of essential fatty acids in children manifest themselves as cases of: asthma, eczema, dry skin and excessive thirst.

Researchers have theorized that children who have hyperactivity disorders may not only be lacking in essential fatty acids, but even if they have sufficient, because of their condition, they may have difficulty metabolizing them into prostaglandins which are essential to help brain communication.

Essential fatty acids are essential for proper brain development, and form a significant part of the structure of brain cell membranes. Low levels of essential fatty acids are frequently linked to reduced levels of intelligence. It is often theorized that this is the reason why children by the age of seven, who were breast-fed as babies, have been shown to have a higher IQ.

Breast milk contains DHA—an essential omega-3 fatty acid, which is critical for brain development. EPA, another important omega-3 essential fatty acid, has been shown in studies to be beneficial for children with dyslexia.

Various studies have highlighted that an elevated intake of essential fatty acids and especially omega-3 fatty acids improves intelligence, reduces aggression and enhances mood.

The richest sources of EPA and DHA are oily fish such as salmon, tuna, mackerel and herring's. These fish are also rich in another component of brain nutrients—phospholipids. Interestingly, the brain and nervous system of a fetus uses up more than half the available nutrients in the mothers body during its development in the womb.

The brain is very reliant on glucose, with roughly half the glucose in the body driving it. It is also dependent on essential fats and phospholipids. Research in the United Kingdom has highlighted that a woman's brain shrinks during pregnancy.

It is known that it is the size of the cells in the brain—not the number that changes. It is theorized that the fetus draws off supplies of essential fats and phospholipids from the mother if insufficient are available. If the theory proves correct, then this demonstrates how important it is to make sure that there are adequate quantities of these essential brain nutrients for both the mother and the fetus.

Essential Fatty Acids and the Vitamin and Mineral Link

As just discussed, there is a tendency for children with hyperactive disorders to have difficulty converting essential fatty acids into prostaglandins; this is the result of children being intolerant to possibly gluten and dairy products. Not only that, but conversion is often restricted by inadequate amounts of different vitamins and minerals which are required by various enzymes for the transition process. Included in this group are such things as vitamin B3, B6, and vitamin C, biotin, zinc and magnesium. Researchers discovered some time ago that a zinc deficiency is not unusual in children who have learning difficulties.

I would recommend that your children eat oily fish at least three times a week and a daily portion of seeds to ensure they get a good level of essential fatty acids to help their brains develop and boost IQ. On the other hand, if your children do not like fish, and don't take seeds every day, then it is wise to supplement the diet with essential fatty acid supplements.

Try to obtain one that contains GLA (Omega-6), DHA and EPA omega-3. As mentioned previously, Omega-3 EPA is derived from oily fish. You can get Omega-6 from flax seed oil, which is processed from the flax plant. The flax plant is very versatile. Not only is it a rich source of Omega-6 essential fatty acids, but it is also used to produce linen for such things as bed sheets, as well as linseed oil which is used in the paint industry. Flax seed oil is also rich in the Omega-3 essential fatty acids as well.

Children and Supplements

Starting a child on a supplement program can commence as soon as they are no longer being breast-fed. During the breast-feeding time, it is the mother who needs to take the supplements to ensure that she is getting adequate nutrition to fulfil not only her body needs, but the needs of her baby as well.

You can commence adding supplements to a child's diet when they start to consume more solid food rather than breast milk. This is often around the age of six to nine months.

What are the Right Supplements for Children

Many companies have a multi-vitamin and Multi mineral supplement designed for children that contains all the necessary nutrients. You'll find that either solid tablets, a chewable variety or a liquid formula are available. Which one you choose will depend on your child's preferences.

It is a good idea to let your child take their supplements with breakfast. Do not let them take them last thing at night as the B. vitamins especially can have a mild stimulatory effect.

There is also the question of toxicity whereby children are more susceptible than adults to vitamin toxicity. It is therefore wise to work within the doses listed on the label. These doses are designed to ensure that no toxic limits are exceeded. It is not a good idea to give your child more than the recommended levels unless you first consult a qualified naturopath.

12. Equine Therapy

To help children with their autistic condition various forms of therapy are essential. Equine therapy or hippotherapy (the Greek word for horse) as it is sometimes referred to as had a profound impact on many autistic children.

Horse-back riding helps an autistic child achieve a level of self-control, self-confidence, and an awareness of the function of their bodies. In addition, it also helps to focus their concentration in addition to their socializing skills. It also helps them exercise patience, improve their communication skills, helps coordinate hand and eye movements and motor (nerve) skills.

From a physical standpoint horse-back riding can help improve a child's balance in addition to strengthening and tightening muscles.

By using equine therapy a child gains the trust of a horse due to their natural acceptance ability. The child grooms the horse by brushing it, and in addition learns to control the horse. In turn the horse relaxes the child. A bond is formed between the child and the horse; this is something which an autistic child has difficulty in accomplishing. This gives the child a great sense of accomplishment. A child appreciates this interaction with the horse and the benefits it gives them while at the same time they are having some fun.

In the beginning this is a new experience for the autistic child and because they don't like change in their routine the possibility that they will initiate some of their autistic symptoms is quite likely. As the child learns to trust the horse and its movements their autistic symptoms will decline.

Riding a horse is very stimulating to an autistic child and another benefit is often that spontaneous speech will erupt from the child due to excitement that being with the horse generates within them. Over time they will frequently make eye contact with the horse. This eye contact will often transfer to making eye contact with humans, which is something that has not been possible previously.

There are two benefits in using equine therapy; these are developing a physical benefit and a developmental benefit. When riding a horse, a saddle is often not used. Many different riding positions are adopted in order to involve different parts of the body. Correlating movements and senses is something that autistic children have difficulty in achieving, and riding a horse will often make significant improvements in all parts of the body.

If you feel that your child would benefit from equine therapy, then it is a good idea to consult your child's doctor, and for you to research the benefits that your child will gain by pursuing this activity.

13. Ritualistic Behavior

Children and adults who suffer from many different disabilities will often have the tendency to perform ritualistic behaviors which therapists believe are a calming influence on the individual.

Research suggests that the basal ganglia and frontal area of the brain are implicated in the development of repetitive behaviors. Research also suggests that there is a neuropathological link between obsessive compulsive disorder (OCD) and autism.

Various studies have been conducted to try and compare the development of ritualistic behaviors in individuals who either suffer from autism or OCD. And while these behaviors are similar at an early stage of development, over time the similarity appears to serve a different function in the two types. This research has been helpful in providing treatment protocols that could work in children and adults who have autism.

Whilst children with autism, on the surface, will appear to have excellent muscle tone and a normal physical development, they will often portray repetitive and ritualistic behavior that may sometimes be referred to as stereotypic movement disorder. Another common term for this condition is self-stimulation or 'stimming'.

These repetitive motions are referred to in this way as they stimulate the brain—something that the autistic child finds comforting.

Researchers have several theories concerning these behavior patterns and what purpose they serve, or why they are so prevalent in people who suffer from autism. One theory suggests that there is an under-stimulation of the nervous system, and by undertaking these ritualistic behaviors, this is a way of providing stimulus to the nervous system. The theories then go on to suggest that by over stimulating the nervous system, this then provides a normalizing action.

Other typical actions of ritualistic behavior can include: grinding of teeth, waving of hands, rocking movements and nail biting. In some instances these ritualistic actions can be self-harming to the person. Extreme ritualistic actions can include such things as banging the head against a solid object, biting oneself or trying to tear out the skin.

An additional ritualistic behavior can involve language. This action is called echolalia which is defined as the repetition of a single word or phrase. This is something that can be done repetitively or it may be done at specific times of day and for a specific number of times.

A behavior that does not cause self-injury to the individual or others can often be ignored, although it may be irritating and stressful to a person on the receiving end. However, should the behavior be causing self-injury, or the activity is so severe that it cannot be ignored, to the extent that it interferes with an individual's ability to interact with his or her own environment, then this may be addressed by using applied behavioral analysis, sensory stimulation therapy, or medication. It will all depend on what is causing the behavioral pattern.

A child performing ritualistic behaviors in many cases forms part of the basis for an autistic diagnosis. These ritualistic behaviors are something that parents will have to learn to deal with. They can be stressful and irritating at times.

By helping the parents learn how to cope with these situations, and in turn the parents helping their children, those with mild to moderate autism are often able to integrate into society without additional problems.

14. Coping and Support

When parents have a child who has been diagnosed with autism, they will soon discover that it will have a profound effect in the way that the family as a whole interacts with other people; in particular, how the siblings will be treated in school, and looking to the future, how this can impact on the retirement plans of the parents.

Psychologists have known for a long time that stress within the family unit can often be relieved by the parents of an autistic child enlisting the support of family, friends and other people who are in the same situation as they are.

Local support groups can also be a great help as they will make the parents realize that other people are having the same stresses and strains on their family life that they are experiencing. They will also be able to get advice and possibly help in dealing with problems that they are facing at home.

A support group will also be able to give information and advice on what to expect as a child grows and develops. Bear in mind that the symptoms are often different in each child, while the overall diagnosis is still the same, therefore the advice and help on offer will still be relevant.

It is also possible to use a support group to locate good physicians and therapists as well as treatment protocols that will be helpful in treating a child.

Often times living with a child with autism can be a very stressful experience. The stress can also cause other difficulties within the family. Various issues can arise such as personality changes in the siblings, to the parents themselves having relationship issues, and also the onset of health related diseases in the parents and children.

Health issues can include heart disease, stroke, diabetes, anxiety disorders and a compromised immune system, which can mean that individuals in the family unit can be more susceptible to colds and other illnesses.

The number of children being diagnosed with autism in the United States is rising steadily according to the Centers for Disease Control and Prevention (CDC). They estimate that one in 88 children has an autism spectrum disorder. That is an increase from one in 150 just 10 years ago.

These rising numbers can have a stressful impact on finding suitable support groups and help in the local area. Parents shouldn't try to cope on their own. If they do, they will only increase the stress within the family unit.

Once it has been accepted that help and support is needed a good place to start is at the local hospital by asking the social worker about local support groups. The majority of hospitals are aware of what support groups are available in the area and who to contact.

If the local hospital can't help, then try the local chapter of the national organization who will be able to put you in touch with other families who are having the same experiences.

While support groups are important it is always helpful to find a family whom parents can talk to on a personal basis. This can be extremely useful in helping to reduce stress and also having someone else to call upon in times of emergency.

Support at School

It is the right of all parents who have children with autism to have school support in all school settings. Interestingly, it is often found that there are more children enrolled in school with autism than many people realize. Most children with autism go to public schools where they are mainstreamed into the public school system.

Each child with autism has very specific needs. The schooling they will receive should be adapted to the individual needs of the child. Some children with autism may require one-on-one support systems, but they will still attend public school. Some children may attend half-day classes in a special needs environment, followed by half a day in a regular classroom. An alternative is for a child to attend a special school for autistic children. Whatever education path you choose to follow, it is a very personal choice.

If you decide to choose a public school for your child he or she will be integrated into a "normal" school environment where a group of people will work with your child based on that child's individual needs. It is important to understand, that in this scenario your child will just receive an "adequate" education. This is fine if you're happy with this arrangement. It is also important to remember that your child will be around children without autistic problems. But in reality there may be other special needs children in attendance with possibly the same symptoms as your own child.

Another option is to enrol your autistic child in a private school for autistic children. This way, your child will be with other children who have a similar condition. Your child will receive special attention and often specific resources are available for a child with autism. Programs will be individualized and geared to each child's needs. It is important to bear in mind that your child will be with children who have similar condition to your child, which may or may not be a good idea. Enrolling a child in a private school can be really expensive.

A further option that many parents choose is home-schooling. Your child will get their education in a familiar home setting. You are often the best judge as to what abilities your child has and you are then able to adapt their schooling needs to their abilities.

In a home-schooling environment it is also important to be mindful that social interaction is also a beneficial part of learning.

It is a very personal matter which school system you choose for your child. It is important to base this decision on your personal beliefs and what you feel is important for your child. It is also important to bear in mind what goal path you have in mind for your child, and what your child may hope to accomplish.

At the end of the day, you have to make the choice and reach a decision that you will be comfortable with. It is a good idea to ask advice of your child's pediatrician before making a final decision. As a responsible parent, in making these decisions, you are making the wisest possible choices for your child so that they will get the best education that will be right for them.

In Summary

Autism seems to be on the increase in children. Looking at the statistics published by the Centers for Disease Control and Prevention (CDC) makes alarming reading. They estimate that one in 88 children now have an autistic condition which is up from one in 150 just ten years ago.

I find this statistic quite alarming, and like many other diseases of the Western world—it seems to be on the increase. But what can be causing this increase? There are many theories being investigated, but as yet, no definitive answers.

I do think in many cases that the Western diet which is high in fat, sugar, refined carbohydrate, artificial colors, and preservatives and low in fiber is implicated in some way. In addition, I also think that all the fizzy drinks which are high in sugar, chemicals, and in some—caffeine are also involved in some way.

When I was researching for one of my books, I noted that where one of these drinks is put in an aluminum can the chemicals can react against the aluminum with the result that aluminum particles finish up in the drink, which then is consumed by someone. This then becomes part of heavy metal toxicity—something which can have a very detrimental effect on some of the major organs of the body.

And just reading about that, and all the other things that many people who live in the Western world do to their bodies, makes me believe that many of the diseases that afflict people of all ages is a lot to do with diet and lifestyle.

I've tried to make this book as easy to read as possible, as autism, like many other conditions can be mystifying to the uninitiated.

I have written this book primarily for parents of young children, however, sections of the book are probably more for adults than children. As I was writing this book it seemed to evolve this way, as I realized that adults, who may have been struggling with an autistic condition throughout their life, may get some good benefits by reading it. This book is also intended for those who wish to get a better understanding of what autism is, and as a result, they will be better informed of what an autism sufferer is going through.

About The Author

Brian B Jacques started in business at a young age, and over the ensuing years, he has developed several very successful businesses. But his main interest for the past 40 years has been in natural health research and publishing.

Brian has presented seminars worldwide on such diverse subjects as Health Related issues, Motivation and Personal Development. In addition he has written numerous books, newsletters and articles on these subjects.

His very popular series of Mini Health Books has circulated widely around the world, and many more titles are in preparation.

Brian is a highly motivated individual, so much so that in 1985 he received a UK Industrial Society award for his work in the Motivation and Personal Development fields.

Brian has the following mottos:

- If something does not work out for you, then don't give up, but keep trying, trying, trying until finally you succeed.

- Success or failure in any endeavor is in your own hands.

Brian and his wife divide their time between East Yorkshire, UK and Florida, USA.

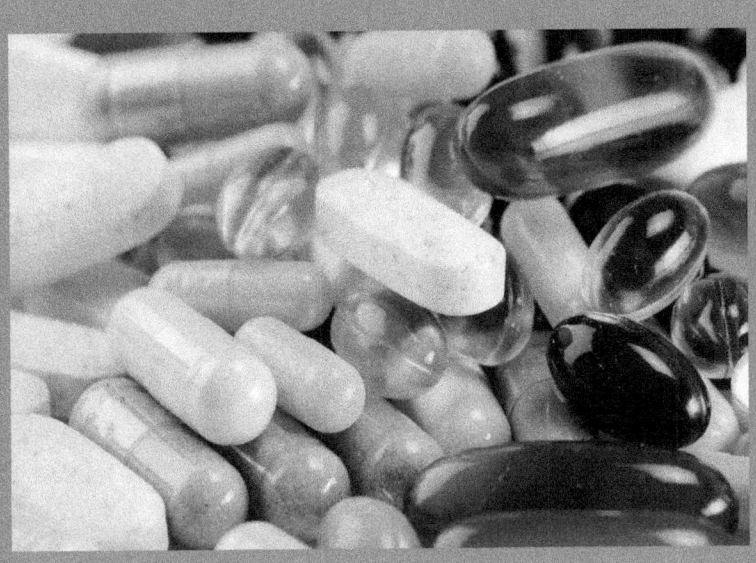